I0411330

Weight Loss Journey:

How a Middle Aged Man Lost Weight, Kept It Off, and Radically Improved His Fitness

- And How You Can Too

By Sunil Tanna

Copyright © 2012 Sunil Tanna

All rights reserved.

ISBN: 1481815598
ISBN-13: 978-1481815598

Weight Loss Journey:

How a Middle Aged Man Lost Weight, Kept It Off, and Radically Improved His Fitness

- And How You Can Too

Copyright & Other Notices

Published in 2012 by Answers 2000 Limited

Copyright © 2012, Sunil Tanna

Sunil Tanna has asserted his right to be identified as the author of this Work in accordance with the Copyright, Designs, and Patents Act 1988.

The author of this work is **not** a doctor or medical professional. This book is **not** intended as medical advice. Readers are advised to see their doctor, should they need treatment for any disease or condition. Readers are also advised to see their doctor before making changes to their diet, exercise regimen, or lifestyle.

Answers 2000 Limited is a private limited company registered in England under company number 3574155. Address and other information about information about Answers 2000 Limited can be found at www.ans2000.com

Latest news & updates from the author can be found at http://www.suniltanna.com/weightloss

Introduction

I was fat, I was unfit, and I was over 40.

It wasn't so bad – I had a beautiful wife, a comfortable home, a decent standard of living, and a loving extended family, including two wonderful nephews. My wife and I longed for a child, unfortunately that hadn't happened, but apart from that, life was pretty good.

Physically however things were heading downhill.

We had moved to the area a few years earlier, and had changed doctor as a result. At my initial check-up with the nurse, I was surprised to learn that my blood pressure was only just short of falling into the high category. The nurse had gently suggested that I really shouldn't have this problem at my age, and that losing some weight would help. She had advised me to make a return appointment to specifically address these issues. However, I half convinced myself that it was most likely an erroneous reading, and even if correct, it wasn't so bad, since I was only at the boundary – not over it. In any case, I didn't go back to nurse.

I was also embarrassed by photographs of me – especially ones taken when I was at the beach. I tried to convince myself that the camera adds a few pounds, but I never could quite explain why it added so many more pounds to me than anybody else.

It wasn't that I hadn't tried diets or doing a bit more

exercise. I had tried several – my problem was that I hadn't stuck with them. I'd either never get properly started, or if I did I'd lose a few pounds while on the program, I would immediately gain them back when I stopped.

In my mind, the problem wasn't that serious. I liked to think that I was only carrying a few extra pounds, and was still almost as fit and healthy as I had been in my youth. I still fancied doing the active physical things that I had done in my younger years, like playing football ("soccer" to my American readers), although, of course, I wasn't doing them. I even emailed a couple of local amateur football clubs hoping to see if I could play.

The truth was I was seriously overweight. In my heart, I knew it. But I didn't like the truth, so I hid from the truth and told myself another story. I had even stopped weighing myself, because frankly I didn't want to know the number. Looking back, I believe my maximum weight was comfortably over 18 stone – 252 pounds (114 kg) – but the truth is I am not precisely sure of the exact figure.

Now, just a few years later (I am 43 at the time of writing), I'm close to my ideal weight (I now weigh around 182 pounds – 83kg) , fitter than I probably have ever been, regularly play competitive sport, and have participated in quite a few demanding physical challenges. I've participated in cross-country runs, including some dressed as Santa Claus (to raise funds for charity). I've also completed, twice, the Bournemouth to Boscombe sea swim – an annual event that involves swimming from one pier to the other, a distance of about 1.5 miles (2.5km), in the very cold waters of the English Channel. And I've completed the Nuts Challenge, an extremely demanding 5.5 mile (8.9km) cross-country assault course, in a quite respectable time. Most importantly of all, I feel fit and healthy.

How did I do it? That of course is what this book is about. When I set out on my weight loss journey, I didn't start with a plan. I discovered things along the way that helped me. Some of it was serendipity – the right things came along at the right time to keep me going.

Can you do it too? That's up to you. If they want it enough, I believe most people can lose excess weight, and improve their general fitness and health. It's partly a matter of determination, and it's partly a matter of knowing how to approach things.

I'm **not** going to give you a diet plan ("eat this for this meal"), and I'm **not** going to give you an exercise plan ("do this on this day"). My experience is that it's really hard to stick to rigid diet or exercise plans. In any case, they only work for the weeks or months when you're actually following them – as soon as you resume your normal life, the weight starts coming back.

Instead, in this book, I want to talk about how you can change your normal life. I will show you what worked for me, including a few things that I discovered purely by dumb blind luck (and if you don't get equally lucky, you probably would otherwise never discover). I also hope to show you how I learned to think about these issues and how I believe you should too, so that you can **permanently** keep the weight off.

There are a few things that I should finally make 100% clear before proceeding:

1. I am **not** a doctor, **nor** am I a health professional. I have absolutely no specialist knowledge or training on such matters.

2. This book is **not** intended as medical advice. If you want medical advice, or need treatment for any disease or condition, please go and see your doctor.

3. I would strongly advise you to go and see your doctor before making changes to your diet or lifestyle. This especially applies if contemplating taking up vigorous forms of exercise, for the first time, or after a gap of many years.

4. I can only tell you about what worked for me. Your experiences may vary from mine. Hopefully I can give you some ideas about how to change your lifestyle and ways of thinking that will help you, but in the end, it's up to you.

Recognizing Where You Truly Stand

I suspect most people who are overweight are at least a little like I was.

The weight has accumulated over the years, the change has been gradual, and they think of themselves as being just a few pounds over where they should be. If they were fit and active in their younger years, they don't necessarily see themselves as being vastly different, even if their body currently feels completely different.

Perhaps they don't look at the bathroom scales anymore?

Perhaps they convince themselves that their holiday photographs are simply "unflattering" rather than showing the truth?

If they do look at their weight, and put it into a BMI Calculator, perhaps they convince themselves that the reason they are fall into the overweight or obese range, is that they have a large frame or muscular body.

Do you recognize yourself in any of these descriptions?

In my case, all these were true at different times, but I only came to realize the extent of my weight problem gradually, over a period of time, and after a couple of wake-up calls. The truth is that I wish I had come to grips with it sooner.

The first wake-up call was the visit to the nurse that I've

already described. While I said that I never went back to nurse, what I didn't mention previously was that I eventually had to go back to the same doctor's surgery to get a prescription for antibiotics after getting a chest infection. The doctor saw my notes, and decided to measure my blood pressure again – it was still borderline high. It was getting harder to hide from the truth.

The second wake-up call was when I got a response to one of my emails to local football (soccer) clubs. They invited me to attend one of their training sessions. I desperately wanted to play, but I knew I wasn't up to it, so made an excuse not to go. Fortunately for me, I was invited again a little while later, and this time I did go.

It was a boiling hot day in August. Even though I was sweating terribly, I was embarrassed at how unfit I looked, and I kept my tracksuit and hooded-sweatshirt on for the entire training session. The training session should not have been difficult – a little light jogging around a field, kicking a ball around in some exercises, and a short practice game. Other members of the club, many in their 40s, and some in their 50s, none of them professional athletes, completed the session without any difficulty. I however severely struggled to keep going (although, perhaps by luck, I somehow did manage to score a goal in the practice game), and was in physical pain for more than a week afterwards. I actually remember going to Brighton beach several days later, and struggling to walk up the beach because of the pain in my legs.

I could no longer hide from it. I could no longer lie to myself that I was "slightly out of condition", or "just carrying a few extra pounds". I had to face the facts. I was overweight, my fitness was terrible, and I needed to do something about it.

Even then, it took a while for me to fully admit just how overweight and unfit I was, but I eventually set myself goals of losing weight and improving my fitness, and I believe you can too. The first step is to figure out where you really stand, which direction you are heading, and where you need to get to.

1. You need to know how much you weigh

People lie, even to themselves, but numbers don't lie.

Get a decent pair of scales (throw out those worn-out old mechanical scales which can gain or lose 10 pounds depending on which way you are leaning). You don't have to spend a fortune – a digital bathroom scale, is not expensive, and should give consistent results (results should not vary by more than 1 or 2 pounds if you take several measurements). And make sure you put your new set of scales on a hard and level surface such as your tiled bathroom floor.

You also need to get in the habit of weighing yourself,

consistently, every single day.

I would strongly recommend weighing yourself once first thing in the morning as soon as you get up, and once last thing at night, in both cases with no clothes on. Your weight for the day is simply the average of the two numbers – add them together and divide by two. I don't know whether this method more accurately measures your "true weight" than any other method, but what I have found, is that it keeps down the amount of random variation, and provides a relatively consistent basis for doing day-to-day comparisons.

2. Keeping Track

I found it best to jot down my weight in a notebook each time I measured it. Your memory might be better than mine, but in my case it was the only way I could remember the night-time number by the following day.

Each day your weight might go up or down due to random variations, but in the long-run you should hopefully see a trend in the right direction.

If you want to, you can even use spreadsheet software to chart your progress, and if you're statistically inclined, you could even calculate all sorts of statistics like 7-day moving averages for your weight, but, strictly speaking, none of that kind of stuff is really necessary. Just look at this month's numbers, and compare them to those of a month or two ago – if you're losing weight, they should generally be a few pounds lower.

For those readers who are interested, although as I said it's not strictly necessary, I have put a spreadsheet (suitable for use in Microsoft Excel or Apache OpenOffice) on my website at http://www.suniltanna.com/weightloss . My spreadsheet calculates your daily average weight, and once you have entered enough data, your moving average weight for the last 7 days, and how much you have lost (or gained) since last month.

3. Setting Yourself a Goal

BMI stands for "Body Mass Index". It's a crude measure, expressed in a single number, of whether you are underweight, overweight, obese, or in the normal range. The ideal healthy BMI is generally considered to be in the range 18.5 to 25.0.

You can look up more details of BMI at http://en.wikipedia.org/wiki/Body_mass_index

There are many websites offering free online BMI calculators, where you can type in your height and weight, and instantly get the result back. I've posted links to some BMI calculators (and some other BMI information) on my website at http://www.suniltanna.com/weightloss. Alternatively, you can simply try searching for "BMI calculator" into Google.

You probably have read that BMI is a very crude measure, and doesn't work for everybody. For example, most heavily muscled Olympic athletes are classified, according to BMI, as being overweight or obese, despite the fact they have very low body-fat percentages.

So if you are overweight, it's easy to convince yourself that your BMI isn't expressing the true facts about your situation. You can easily attribute your high BMI to an unusual body-shape, a large frame, a muscular upper-body or legs, etc. When I was overweight, I did that myself, attributing at least part of my high BMI to my large frame, broad shoulders, and fairly chunky arms and legs.

If your body is rock-hard and you already look like an Olympic decathlete, then maybe you can discard BMI. Likewise, if you ask your doctor and he says that BMI doesn't apply to you, then take his advice.

But otherwise, my suggestion is that you at least start with the assumption that BMI might be more or less correct in your case.

If you feel flabby, if you have visible fat on your stomach, arms, or legs, or if you have love handles, then a high BMI is telling you something. It may not be telling you exactly to the pound, but it is correctly diagnosing you as overweight. Remember, just because BMI doesn't work for everybody, and might not be completely accurate for all body types (including perhaps people like you), BMI's inaccuracy won't magically make your love handles vanish.

So, the next step is to start messing with one of those online BMI calculators.

First, if you haven't done it already, calculate what your current BMI is.

Next, you can try putting in gradually lower hypothetical weights for yourself, until you can reach a BMI of 25 (the upper end of the normal range). If you're seriously overweight, these hypothetical numbers might seem impossibly far away right now.

You may well be saying to yourself something like "Because of my unusually large shoulders and chest, even when I become thin, my BMI will probably be 28". That's okay – if your future hypothetical weight is lower than your current weight (and it should be, because you know you need to lose some flab, right?), then you've set yourself an initial target.

In future, you will be able to see how far you have progressed towards your initial target, by looking at your records of daily weigh-ins. Eventually, as your weight falls, you will begin to see whether you've chosen the right target BMI or not. If, as you approach your target BMI (even if it's over 25), you reach a point when you feel that you don't need to lose any more flab, then you can stick at that weight. On the other hand, if you reach your target BMI, and feel you are still carrying some flab, you can revise your target BMI downwards.

That's exactly what I did. In fact, I did it more than once.

As I said, I have fairly broad shoulders, quite a large frame (my wrists are so large that I've often found it hard to get a watch that fits), and fairly muscular arms and legs (from years of rugby and cross-country runs in school). I therefore convinced myself that my ideal BMI was considerably over 25.

But, each time I reached my then-current target BMI, I found I was still carrying a fair amount of flab.

Right now, I've eliminated most (but not quite all), of the visible flab, and I'm hovering around 25. I guess my target (even with my large frame, broad shoulders, and chunky arms and legs), should have been 24 to 25 all along.

Changing Your Life Permanently

When I realized that I needed to seriously improve my fitness and lose some weight, one of the first things that I thought about was all the diets and exercise programs I had tried before.

None of them had worked.

I won't say that none of them had ever removed a pound. But the problem was that I followed them for a while, gradually lost interest, or got distracted, and then piled the weight back on, usually with a few extra pounds as well.

I realized that if I wanted to lose weight and keep it off, I needed a different approach.

First of all, I needed to change my way of thinking. Instead of following a program for a few weeks or months, losing a bit of weight, and then returning to my old bad habits, I needed to find a way to make **permanent** changes to my eating and exercise habits.

Secondly, and perhaps more importantly, I knew the reason why I hadn't followed previous programs for more than a short-time, and even then, only half-heartedly.

The problem was "friction".

Things which go against the grain of your life have a lot of "friction". If they require you to do things that you don't really want to do (like go hungry), or stop you doing things that you do really want to do (like socializing with family or friends), or which are just tremendously inconvenient, you'll probably find a way not to do them.

It's why people join gyms, and stop going after a few weeks – it's easier to simply go home, if you're tired after a long day at work. And it's one of the main reasons why people don't stick to diets. We all prefer to eat foods that we enjoy, are available, and are easy to get hold of. And when we're hungry and in a rush, unhealthy but convenient fast-food today, and starting the diet tomorrow, doesn't seem like such a bad option.

Having identified the problem, my solution was simple. I needed to find ways to try to reduce the "friction" of doing things that were good for my health or fitness – things like eating the right kind of foods and doing regular exercise – and, where possible, increase the "friction" of doing unhealthy, fattening things.

Once I did that, I gradually found myself doing the right things, more and more often, just because it was easier.

Moreover, over a period of time, new habits can get engrained. Many of us walk around the supermarket on autopilot buying the same foods as last week, or choose what to eat without really thinking about it. I discovered that by making doing the right things into a routine, eventually they became habitual – for example, when shopping I'd buy healthy foods without really thinking about them, or when unthinkingly choosing a snack, I'd pick up an apple rather than a bag of potato chips.

I also strongly believe that most people not only follow habitual behaviours, but eventually grow to like them. That at least is my experience. So, if you establish habits of eating healthily, you will actual feel uncomfortable if somebody offers you a greasy plate of fried food. And if you establish a habit of doing daily exercise, you will feel uncomfortable if you do nothing all day.

That is why I am talking about changing your life **permanently**. That is what I aimed to do, and that is what you can do too.

People sometimes ask "When you will you finish your diet?", "When will you go back to eating normally?" (By which they mean, eating unhealthily like I used to), or "When will you finish your exercise program?"

They are usually shocked when I reply "Never."

What they don't understand is that I did **not** "go on a diet". Neither did I "follow an exercise program". I changed my life – and made eating more healthily and taking daily exercise integrated parts of my life. Removing these things from my life (and reverting to my old ways) would take far more effort, than simply continuing with them.

Low Friction Exercise Routines

My wife bought me a static exercise bike as a gift during the year I turned 41. It was actually before I started seriously losing weight – it was when I was still in the stage of thinking "I only need to lose a few extra pounds."

Sometimes you get lucky though, and getting the exercise bike turned out to be a huge stroke of luck for me.

It massively reduced the amount of effort needed to maintain daily exercise as part of my life.

Yes, I have since got into running and swimming, and cycling outdoors, and lots of other things, but the static bike is always there, available for me to use, in my own home, whenever I want to.

I can jump on the bike and pedal away, no matter what the weather is like outside. Even if I am snowed in and unable to leave the house (which has happened a couple of times, as we seem to have exceptionally hard Winters in the last couple of years), I can still manage to do some vigorous exercise.

Moreover since the bike is always in my house, and is kept in an accessible location (despite my wife's objections it remains in the living room), there is no friction stopping me from using it regularly. If I want to get 30 minutes exercise, I don't have to spend an additional 30 minutes driving to and from the gym or the swimming pool. And I don't even have to miss my favourite TV programs!

I can't recommend using a static exercise bike highly enough (although it did take me quite a while to get used to the saddle), but other options you could consider are a treadmill or a rowing machine. The real point is that I urge you to find some kind of exercise that you can do in your own home, and which you will do, even if you are tired, or if your car is being repaired, or if there's a blizzard outside. Yes, you might do other things as well, like go running, swim, or go to the gym, but you want to find something that you can do every single day, without fail, and which ensures you will get a guaranteed minimum amount of regular exercise.

Secondly, when you do get your bike or treadmill or rowing machine, make sure you put in a place where you will use it. It's no good putting in a cold draughty basement which you don't really want to go to – as sooner or later, you will actually stop going there.

You want to put this key piece of exercise equipment in a comfortable location, which you enjoy going to. For most people, I suspect that means the living room, which you may or may not be able to get your partner to agree to. If necessary show your partner this book in order to persuade them of the importance of making your exercise equipment easily accessible. You can also try explaining to your partner that you are going to spend a lot of time exercising, and that you would much rather spend as much time as possible in their presence. But if you really are unable to convince them, you should at least ensure that your alternate location is comfortable, with enough to occupy your mind as well as your body – a TV and DVD player, for example.

Also, if you're planning ahead, your choice of entertainment, should influence your choice of exercise machine. One good feature of a static exercise bike is that it is possible to do other things, even while exercising extremely vigorously. Nowadays I not only watch movies on DVD while pedalling, but also read the newspaper or my Kindle, and even do the cryptic crossword. Your experience may vary, but on a treadmill, I'm capable of watching TV or listening to the radio, but not much else, and on a rowing machine, I could probably listen to the radio, but that would be about it.

Aside from using your main exercise machine, you may also want to find other work-out activities that you can **conveniently** perform in your own home. For example, I have a pair of dumb bells (actually I have several pairs as I've gradually increased the weight) that I often spend 15 or 20 minutes working with while standing in front of the TV.

Competitive Sport as a Motivator

One of the big most motivators for wanting to lose weight and improve my fitness was that I wanted to play regular football (soccer). It's not that I am especially good at football, but I do enjoy the game.

But football has some other attributes that made it ideal for improving fitness:

First of all, it's a physically challenging game – the game itself involves vigorous exercise.

Secondly, it's competitive. The aim is always to play as well as you can, and if possible to win. The teams I play in, don't always win (we probably lose more often than not, as we're often playing against younger and more skilled teams), but we always try hard.

Thirdly, it's a regular commitment: I currently play in two 5-a-side football teams, as well as occasional 11-a-side football. The 5-a-side teams play almost every week of the year, either on all-weather surfaces, or in an indoor sports hall, so there is no extended break from the game in which to get unfit again.

Of course, not everybody reading this guide is going to say "I love football". In fact, I expect most of my readers will not be particularly interested in playing football. My point is however that you can look for a sport that shares some of the attributes that football has for me – vigorous, competitive, and played regularly.

If you like team sports, check your local sports centres, and you can also look on the Internet (including websites like Gumtree) for teams that are looking for players. You could even consider starting your own team – for example, by phoning the local leagues to ask if they have details of any unattached players, putting an advert on Gumtree or in the sports centre, etc.

Likewise, if you enjoy tennis or squash, you could take one of these up. But don't just play for laughs or go for a few lessons – join a league, and commit yourself to playing regularly, and trying to win in a competitive environment (it doesn't matter so much whether you actually win or lose – it's simply important that you try your hardest to win).

Even in solo sports like swimming or running, you can introduce a competitive element – you simply have to compete against yourself. Count laps when swimming, or follow a standard route when running, and see if you can go further and/or faster in less time. The key is that you have to push yourself a little bit – not so hard as to do yourself an injury – but enough so that you can both face a challenge, and gradually improve your fitness.

Big Hairy Audacious Goals

I first read about Big Hairy Audacious Goals ("BHAGs" for short, pronounced "bee-hags") in a business book, "Built to Last", by Jim Collins and Jerry Porras. Essentially, they were ambitious goals that various companies set themselves, which were beyond the limit of what most people thought possible at the time.

Some examples, were Jack Welch at General Electric aiming to be number 1 or number 2 in every single market in which the company competed, Sam Walton aiming to double the number of Wal-Mart stores and massively increase sales volume in 10 years, IBM building the revolutionary 360 mainframe computer, and Boeing entering the market for large commercial aircraft (culminating in building the largest commercial jet then imaginable, the 747 Jumbo Jet).

The purpose of such BHAGs was that they served as a focus for the organization, and made the entire company stretch to achieve seemingly impossible results.

In terms of improving my fitness and health, I have found that setting myself similar BHAGs has served as both focus and motivation for me, and helped me achieve things that I once would not have thought possible.

I've participated in Santa Dashes (cross-country runs dressed as Santa Claus) twice. The first time I did it, I wasn't sure if I would be able to complete the course. I put in lots of extra training before hand to make sure that I really could run the distance. Even with all the training, I have to admit I did struggle to run all the way without stopping. A year later, I did another Santa Dash, without any special training before hand, and I sailed through it. In fact, I am now able to run this kind of distance any time I want, and do quite regularly. What was once a BHAG, has gradually become easy.

Another example, perhaps my first really challenging BHAG, was doing the Bournemouth to Boscombe swim. This is a 1.5 mile (2.5 km) swim in the sea from Bournemouth to Boscombe pier, in the English Channel. I don't want to exaggerate the difficulty, but for me, it was a tough and scary challenge.

The first time I participated, I was nervous. I had trained really hard in the swimming pool, and in the sea when on vacation in Cyprus, but practising in a warm pool or the Mediterranean Sea is not the same as swimming in the cold English Channel. So, I was worried that I might not be able to finish the swim.

It turned out however that I was able to complete the swim relatively easily – I actually had trained so hard that my fitness level far exceeded what was needed to complete this BHAG.

Food & Shopping

I am not an expert on nutrition, or anything like that, so I am not going to tell you exactly what to eat or tell you how to draw-up a diet plan. You probably already know that you should eat a balanced diet, with all the essential vitamins and minerals, but if you don't, you can ask your doctor to explain, or look up this information on any number of government health websites.

Before we start talking about particular foods or eating strategies, I should also say that I firmly believe that the simplest way to lose weight is to concentrate on calories. Some diet plans say that you should eat only certain foods or combinations of food, or pay close attention to what you eat at what time of day. I'm not in a position to say whether such claims are right or wrong, but what I can say is that I find such rigid rules to be impossible to follow.

My simple theory is instead to focus on the amount of calories you burn, and the amount of calories that you take in. If you burn more calories than you take in, then you should lose weight. Of course I have not read all the scientific evidence for or against this theory, but all I can say is that it worked for me.

It apparently also worked (albeit in a way that I would **never** want to try myself, and would **not** recommend to others) for Mark Haub, a nutrition professor at Kansas

State University, who was able to lose weight by eating less calories, despite the fact that those calories came in the form of Twinkies, chips, and sugary snacks. Of course, Mark Haub didn't achieve his weight loss by just eating any amounts of those kinds of foods – he had to use **extremely strict** portion control – but the point is, reducing his calorie intake did help him lose weight. I've posted some links to the Mark Haub related news stories and opinions on my website at http://www.suniltanna.com/weightloss.

Anyway, I've already talked about finding low friction ways of increasing the amount of calories that you burn through exercise, but if you want to lose weight, I believe that it's equally important that you find low friction ways of eating less calorific foods.

The first thing I would do is ask myself "What do I **really** want from my food?"

Here's my list – I suspect yours is likely to be practically identical:

1. I want it to be available when I am hungry.

2. I want it to be convenient. For example, if I am in a rush, I don't have to spend a lot of time obtaining or preparing it.

3. I want it to be tasty and enjoyable to eat.

4. I want it to be filling and satisfying – so I don't

immediately feel hungry again after eating.

You will notice that sweet, sugary, high fat, high calorie, etc. did not appear anywhere on the list.

I firmly believe one of the major reasons why most people eat too many chocolates, candies, salted snacks, junk foods, and other high calorie foods, is simply because they are always immediately available, and they have become, convenient, low friction, options.

In terms of taste, it's true that we might enjoy some of these foods, but the chances are there are many others that we eat purely out of habit or laziness. Even among unhealthy foods that you think you "enjoy", are you really sure that's just not familiarity? Is it possible that you have simply trained yourself to "enjoy" them, and could train yourself not to?

You might be surprised... My own personal experience is that after a few months cutting out the junk completely, there are many junk foods that I once enjoyed that I now find completely unappetizing. That aside, I seriously doubt there are many people who would genuinely say that their go-to junk foods truly are the best things that they've ever tasted.

Finally, I wanted to say most junk foods are not satisfying. There's a reason why people say these foods are "more-ish" or "you can't stop" – the reason is if you eat them, you don't quickly get to a point where you are full and satisfied. If you're going to have a snack, wouldn't it be better to choose one which does leave you full and satisfied?

So how do you use this information? The answer is to change the kinds of food that you keep in your house, and change the way you shop and eat. Make eating healthy low-calorie foods into the low friction option. Eventually eating this way will become a habit, and you'll do it without thinking.

So, first of all, throw out all the junky snacks. If they are not easily available in your own home, you are far less likely to eat them.

Secondly, when you shop, you need to be doing it in a different way. Instead of racing down the usual aisles, throwing the usual things into your trolley, go down every single aisle. Read the labels on packets especially the calorie count (I've put some notes on reading labels below). Try to find the lowest calorie options. Also try to select as much fresh fruit and vegetables (but not potatoes) as possible.

You can also try expanding your horizons – most large supermarkets are constantly introducing new items into their ranges, including types of food that you may never have tasted, such as exotic items influenced by foreign cuisines. Read the labels, and if they are low calorie, don't be afraid to try new things. Why not try to find one new food to try every time you do a large supermarket shop?

It will take some time and effort, especially on your first few shopping expeditions, but you should eventually be able to identify a set of lower calorie, healthier options, that you can eat on a regular basis.

You also need to be realistic in shopping. For example, if you enjoy a mid-morning snack, or a snack watching TV in the evening, you probably aren't going to cut that habit out. Instead set yourself an achievable goal – eating only healthy snacks - and keep some healthy snacking items available, which you can eat at these times.

Likewise, you might know that you don't usually have time or energy to prepare a cooked dinner from scratch on a weekday evening. You don't want a greasy takeaway or a super high-calorie cheesy pizza from your freezer to be the fall-back option. Keep some easy-to-prepare low calorie options in your fridge or freezer – even if these are microwavable ready-meals from the supermarket's healthy range, they are better than eating a greasy slab of dough with a two-inch thick layer of industrial by-product cheese on the top.

Reading Labels

One of the most important aspects of improving your shopping habits is **carefully** reading the labels.

You don't just need to read the large print on the front

of the packet, but read the actual calorie number, which is usually hidden on the back. Just because something is labelled as "low calorie" or "healthy" in large print on the front of the packet, that doesn't necessarily mean it actually is!

The calorie numbers are often expressed in either "calories per serving", or per 50g or 100g of weight. In such cases, you need to think about what these labels actually mean in terms of what you are going to eat. In my experience, the amount of food in a "serving", or a 50g or 100g portion, is often far less than I would ever be likely to eat.

I've come across relatively small microwavable ready-meals which say in very large print something like "350 calories", but in much smaller print "contains 2 servings", or even "contains 3 servings". Given that I would be likely to eat a whole ready-meal, it really means 700 or 1,050 calories – which isn't such a good number!

Likewise, when calories are expressed per 50g or per 100g, you need to think about what is a realistic portion size for you. I've found that 50g or 100g is nearly always a tiny fraction of what I would actually eat. If the whole packet weighs 500g, and I am likely to eat about one quarter of it in one session, then I need to think of it as not being 188 calories per 50g, but as being a packet of 1,880 calories (that's 10 X 50g, and 10 X 188 calories), which means nearly 500 calories per actual serving (1,880 calories divided 4).

If you think of things this way, you many discover that many foods that you once thought of as being low calorie and not fattening, probably have contributed more to your weight-gain than you previously realized.

In short, the goal is to gradually identify more and more foods, which you enjoy eating, could eat more regularly, and which are lower in calories than the parts of your old diet which they will replace.

Choosing Foods

As I've already said, I am not going to tell you exactly what to eat. I also want to add that neither will I tell you how many calories you should eat.

If you want to lose weight, I believe your goal when choosing foods shouldn't be to precisely count calories, but simply to find healthy foods containing significantly less calories than some of the things that you currently eat. Moreover, your new food choices need to still need to be enjoyable to eat, leave you satisfied and full, and be convenient low friction items that you can easily integrate into your daily life.

In this chapter, I have made suggestions about types of food that you might try having less of (or even eliminate completely from your diet), and others than you might to be able increase. Of course, these are just my suggestions, and you don't have to follow them exactly. The real point is to end-up with a healthier, less calorific diet, that you will enjoy eating.

Bread

Bread can contain quite a lot of calories, and in my experience it doesn't even fill me up. Quite soon after eating a sandwich, I'm hungry for more, and could easily eat another one. Obviously the amount of calories per slice does vary depending on the type of bread, but if there are 80 calories per slice (some sliced bread actually contains more), and you end-up eating 4 or 6 slices, it's a lot of calories even before you count toppings, sandwich fillings, or add any sides to your sandwich.

I should also note that I am of Indian descent, and it's a normal part of an Indian diet to eat various Indian versions of bread with meals. These include as naan, chapatis, and parathas, many of which are either fried, and or coated with ghee (Indian butter).

My solution was simply to eliminate bread, as much as reasonably possible, from my diet. I generally don't eat sliced bread or Indian breads at all – and to be honest, I don't miss them. I have still got a weakness for pita bread when eating at a Greek or Turkish restaurant, but since I don't go to such restaurants too often, it isn't that much of a problem.

Here's how I eliminated most breads from my diet:

1. I no longer eat sandwiches for lunch, but have found other alternatives such as soup, or salads, or low-calorie ready-meals. These are usually more satisfying in any case.

2. When eating Indian meals, I never eat naan, chapatis or parathas, but always have boiled rice instead.

3. For "snacking", when possible I have fruit, or something else entirely different from bread (more on

this later), but other alternatives to bread that I use include: rice cakes, matzo crackers, and No-No flatbread, all of which have a surprisingly low number of calories per piece.

Potatoes

There's a good chance, that like I was, you may be eating far too many potatoes. Fried potatoes (French fries, chips, crisps, etc.) are obviously the worst way to eat potatoes, but you might be getting far too many calories and carbohydrates in other kinds of potatoes too.

I don't know about you, but I don't find potatoes especially filling - I could eat a lot of roast potatoes (for example) before I felt really full. Let's be honest, about it, potatoes are also relatively tasteless – there's a reason why we people eat potatoes with ketchup, or salt and vinegar.

If you want to cut calories, I'd therefore suggest as much as possible, eliminating potatoes from your diet or substituting them for other vegetables, especially green vegetables. Brussel sprouts, cabbage, pak choi (Chinese cabbage), courgette (zucchini), bell peppers, sweet corn, or peas, are all things that you can probably eat more of, to compensate for a reduction in potatoes.

Cheese

Cheese can be a huge source of calories, and when you think about it, it's easy to drastically reduce, or even temporarily eliminate from your diet.

Here are some of the situations where you might encounter cheese, and how you could deal with them:

1. As a snack in itself, for example, "cheese and crackers". Easy – cut it out, don't choose cheese when eating out, and don't keep this snack in your house.

2. In a sandwich filling or in a burger: If you follow my suggestions about bread, you'll probably be eating far less of these anyway. On the rare occasions, when you do have one of these, choose a different lower calorie filling for your sandwich (e.g. ham instead of cheese), or have a burger without cheese.

3. In prepared foods. Some examples include oven-cooked mushrooms with cheese, or melted cheese as a topping on pizza or pasta. This one again is simple: don't choose dishes where cheese is an integral part of item. And remember, pizza or pasta does not have to have cheese on the top – even most takeaway pizza vendors are happy to prepare a thin crust (less bread) pizza with lots of vegetable toppings but no cheese.

4. Where cheese (or a variant of it) is the main part of the dish – such as Indian paneer dishes. You will just have to avoid these ones!

If you really enjoy cheese, these ideas might sound drastic, but trust me; this could well be one of the easiest ways to significantly reduce your calorific intake. Once you've changed your habits, you probably won't even miss cheese – and I can say that speaking as a former-cheese addict!

Finally, if you need an incentive to make you want to abandon cheese simply read the calorie numbers on the cheese packets when shopping. You will be shocked at how many calories even small amounts of cheese can contain.

Milk

Switch to skimmed milk. It might seem watery and tasteless at first, but after a month or two, you should get used to it. Once you do, I expect that you won't want to go back, because if you then ever try semi-skimmed or full-fat again (perhaps when somebody puts some in your tea or coffee), you will find them unpleasantly creamy.

Meat & Fish

Meat, and to a less extent fish, can be high calorific foods.

First of all, I would suggest you try and reduce the

amount of meat that you eat in total:

1. Vegetarian options usually contain fewer calories than meat – so consider trying things like mushroom burgers instead of beef burgers, or Quorn (a popular vegetarian meat substitute) instead of meat. Likewise, when eating out, be sure to take a good look at the vegetarian options available on the menu (vegetarian pizzas, without cheese, can be quite tasty, and Indian restaurants (for example) usually have lots of excellent vegetarian choices). You don't have to become a vegetarian, but it doesn't hurt to eat vegetarian sometimes.

2. Bulk up your meal with healthy vegetables. For example, if you eat lots of Brussel sprouts, you will need less roast chicken!

Of course, unless you are a vegetarian, you will continue to eat meat and fish sometimes. When you do eat meat dishes – try (usually) to choose fish in preference to chicken, and chicken in preference to red meat. Make sure you don't choose fried, bread-crumbed, or pastry-coated meat dishes. And cut off the skin and fat from cuts of meat that you are about to eat.

Fruit & Vegetables

One of the easiest ways to reduce your calorific intake is to increase the amount of fresh fruit and vegetables that you eat.

My experience is that when I eat more vegetables, I need far less highly-calorific meat and potatoes to feel full. You can use this to your advantage both when choosing what meals to eat, and when selecting choosing the items within a meal – for example, if having a roast chicken dinner, trying have less (or no) potatoes, perhaps a little less meat, and compensating by eating more healthy low-calorie green vegetables such as Brussel sprouts.

Another tip is for to look for tasty prepared vegetables that you can incorporate into your meals. For example, most supermarkets in my area sell a "Mediterranean-style" mix of prepared vegetables (containing a mix of chopped courgettes (zucchini), bell peppers, onions, and baby tomatoes, plus herbs), which is tasty, filling, and very easy to cook. Eating this, instead of a side of bread or potatoes, is an easy way to save calories.

Eating more fresh fruit is also an excellent way of reducing your calorific intake. You can eat fruit both with your meals, and use it as a snack food. Obvious choices are apples, oranges, and bananas, but you don't need to limit yourself to these. Most supermarkets offer a wide variety of different fruits, all year round. I particularly enjoy blackberries, blueberries, and strawberries, and have made these regular parts of my diet (I eat a packet of each of them most days).

One thing to watch out for however is fruit juices. They may be tasty and seem healthy, but they are usually extremely sweet and high calorific. If you calculate the number of calories per actual serving (not per "suggested serving"), you might be shocked. It's up to you what you do, but I've pretty much cut fruit juice out my diet completely – I prefer to get my vitamin C from fresh fruit!

Ready-meals

Ready-meals and other ready foods have a bad reputation, because they often are full of calories, and many have excessive amounts of fat, salt, or sugar. Some of this reputation may be deserved, but I don't believe it's true in every case – you need to get in the habit of reading labels.

If you spend some time in the supermarket looking at ready-meals, you soon learn that there is a vast difference between the various types of ready-meals on offer. Even different brand versions of what is supposedly the same dish, may well contain hugely different numbers of calories!

Most large supermarkets offer a healthy-eating or low-calorie range of ready-meals, and there are also well-known brands of ready-meals available. A few items in these ranges may well contain a surprisingly high number of calories (so keep reading the labels), but you should be able to find plenty of choices where the entire ready-meal is just 300 to 400 calories, and even some choices (particularly vegetarian dishes, such as those containing Quorn) which are less than 300 calories.

I don't know about you, but I find a 300 calorie lasagne ready-meal a lot more satisfying and filling than a sandwich at lunch time (and I wouldn't eat two lasagnes, but I might well eat two sandwiches).

Likewise, if you have a ready-meal in the evening sometimes, perhaps accompanied by a packet of Mediterranean-style vegetables, you can get a whole, extremely filling meal in for less than 500 calories (or perhaps slightly more if you eat lots of fruit as your dessert).

In summary, I might not going to advise you to eat ready-meals all the time, but I am going to say – if you shop carefully – and use them on occasion, they can be:

1. Extremely filling and satisfying

2. Helpful in exercising portion control

3. Helpful in limiting (and helping you to know) how many calories you are eating

4. Much better than the other convenience options (such as drive-through fast-food, takeaways, or delivery pizzas) when you're tired or in a rush.

Soups

Soups can be a great addition to your diet, but again you have to shop carefully and read the labels.

If you have time, you can of course make your own soups from scratch, but if not, take a look at the canned varieties. You will find that you have a huge number of options to choose from, many of which you may never have previously tried.

If you look at the 410g cans, in my experience, the label usually describes the number of calories per serving, assuming two servings per can. If you are actually going to have the whole can in one go, you of course need to double this number.

The good news? You can find many soups which have less than 200 calories in an entire 410g can! A can of soup (**without** bread) offers a hot, filling, low calorie lunch option.

Rice & Pasta

Rice and pasta can be quite calorific, so if you eat a lot of them, you might want to reduce your intake somewhat. However, whether you do or not, it's usually possible to reduce the number of calories from such dishes, by eating carefully:

1. When eating rice, choose boiled or steamed rice

instead of fried rice or pilau rice.

2. When eating pasta, don't add cheese, and don't have pasta dishes with creamy sauces.

3. When choosing noodles, choose boiled soup noodles instead of fried noodles.

Incidentally, while probably not ideal in many other ways (they can be quite salty), instant soup noodles (again read the labels and choose widely) can offer a quick, satisfying, and cheap, low-calorie lunch. Boil a kettle and make the noodles, use quite a bit more water than suggested, so as to make a soup, throw in a small packet of cooked prawns (shrimp) and a dash of chilli sauce – instant low-calorie lunch! Using the cheapest noodles from the cheapest local supermarket, and a small packet of cooked prawns (shrimp), I can make a very large and filling bowl of soup with only about 260 calories (151 for the noodles, 109 for the prawns/shrimp).

Breakfast Cereals

Breakfast cereals, even the supposedly healthy varieties, can contain an amazingly large number of calories. This isn't always immediately obvious, because the calorie figures given on the packet are usually given per serving (and without milk or added sugar), and of course, suggested serving sizes are often rather small. 190 calories "per serving", might sound good, until you realize that you are likely to eat 2, 3 or even 4 suggested servings at a stroke.

Here are some ideas to cut down on calories from eating breakfast cereals:

1. First of all, do **not** add sugar, and use skimmed milk.

2. You can try choosing cereals which come in discrete pieces (such as Weetabix or Oatibix) rather than free-flowing cereals where it is hard to limit the portion size.

3. Eat something else for breakfast instead! A 410g can of low-fat rice-pudding, contains around 360 calories, and is an extremely filling and satisfying breakfast. For my own breakfast I usually have a can of low-fat rice-pudding, plus blackberries, blueberries, and/or strawberries. Alternatively, when on vacation (and rice-pudding isn't so easy to find), I usually have 2 bananas and a small (180 calorie) packet of unsalted cashew nuts.

Carbonated Drinks

If you are currently drinking sugary drinks like colas, or lemonades, you need to either eliminate or replace them. They are a huge source of calories.

Some people say that you should stop drinking all carbonated drinks entirely, and switch to water. It sounds like good advice, although I don't know what the latest scientific evidence says. But if you can't eliminate carbonated drinks entirely from your diet (I certainly couldn't do it myself), be sure to **always** drink the diet varieties.

At least in terms of calories (although perhaps not in other ways), diet cola is not at all bad – a 330ml can contains less than 1 calorie, so any realistic amount that you are likely to drink, is not going to make a significant contribution to your calorific intake.

Alcohol

Alcoholic beverages contain a lot of calories as well. Better not to drink them at all, but if you must, limit yourself to one glass of wine, or one can of beer on a Saturday night.

Tip: One way that I have found which can make beer last a little longer is to make shandy (using diet lemonade).

Sugar in Tea or Coffee

Just don't. You'll get used to it.

Fried Foods, Sweets & Cakes

You probably already know that you should not be eating too many of these. But the chances are, like most people, you are probably eating far too much of them.

Cut them out completely if you can. Reduce them drastically if you can't.

It is true that you need some carbohydrate in your diet, but the fact is that you can get it from other sources. Moreover, if you completely stop eating these foods for a while, eventually you may find, like I did, that you no longer find such foods to be nearly so attractive.

Even now, I've been known (but not that frequently – perhaps once or twice while on vacation, or at Christmas) to eat cakes or desserts, but I can honestly say, I often find them unpalatably sweet. As for fried food, it rarely attracts me these days. When I was starting to improve diet, I have to admit, I did allow myself a maximum of one fried dish (usually at a Japanese restaurant) per week, but even that attraction has gradually waned. In short, if you get out of the habit of eating sugary and fried food, I expect that your own desire for it will also gradually disappear.

Meal Ideas

I've already talked about individual foods, so, to a certain extent, this chapter will recap the previous one, however there are a few additional ideas and suggestions that I will add as we go through the day.

Breakfast

Some people say that breakfast is the most important meal of the day, and I think there is some truth in that.

First of all, my experience is that if you skip breakfast, you are far more likely to eat unhealthily as the day goes on. I don't know about you, but if I miss breakfast, by the time 11 O'Clock comes around, I will be starving, and will eat whatever I can without much thought to health or calories.

Another reason why such importance is given to breakfast is that it is supposed to get your metabolism going again, after the night-time slow down. If you skip breakfast, your metabolic rate supposedly stays low for longer, which not only makes you feel sluggish, but also means that you will burn fewer calories during the day. As I've said previously, I'm not a health or nutrition expert, so can't honestly say whether this theory is true, but subjectively, to me at least, it feels like it could be.

So my rule: Always eat breakfast.

So what should you eat or not eat for breakfast?

1. I don't believe that eating a cooked or fried breakfast is a good idea – far too many calories!

2. Bread and toast, as well as bready foods such as waffles, Danish pastries, buns, etc., also all tend to be highly calorific (and in my experience not that filling, anyway) – so again, I would suggest that you try to avoid them if possible.

3. Breakfast Cereals – As already discussed, many cereals contain a lot of calories per actual serving that you are likely to eat (as opposed to per suggested serving). If you are going to eat cereals, and want to keep your calorie intake down, you are going to need to exercise very careful portion control.

4. As I've already mentioned, low-fat canned rice-pudding, turned out to be a very good option for me – around 360 calories for a large satisfying portion (an entire 410g can). Other options you might want to look at include low-fat cans of semolina and tapioca puddings, or low-fat yoghurts. Always be sure to read the labels, as the amount of calories in different brands of these foods can vary widely.

5. Fresh fruit is also a good choice to add to your breakfast – bananas, oranges, blackberries, blueberries, strawberries, etc. But don't add any sugar to them! Sometimes I find blackberries or blueberries quite sour – when that happens, I mix them into my rice pudding.

6. Fruit juices – I've already warned you about the number of calories in them, so beware! In any case, if you are eating a fresh orange, do you really need to drink a glass of orange juice as well?

7. Tea and Coffee – Drink them if you like, but remember no sugar, and always used skimmed milk.

Lunch

A lot of people tend to be busy or mixed up in other things (like work) around lunchtime. As a result, lunch tends to be a meal that we don't pay a lot of attention to, or we maybe even occasionally skip.

I don't think it's a good idea to skip lunch. The reason is basically the same as the main reason not to skip breakfast: If you don't eat lunch, you will get very hungry later in the day, and before you know it, you find yourself fighting back your hunger with unwise food choices. Instead, always eat something for lunch, even if it's just a healthy snack (you can always have another healthy snack in the afternoon).

If you're eating lunch on the go, I think you should try to avoid fast-foods and sandwiches. Fast-food obviously tends to be too high in calories, and, as I've said, sandwiches probably won't leave you feeling really full-up (unless of course you eat lots of sandwiches, or one gigantic sandwich – but those options involve massive amounts of calories).

Instead, my suggestions for quick lunches are to consider, packaged salads (which should be clearly labelled with the number of calories they contain), soups, or low-calorie ready meals. Be honest with yourself – is really too much effort to microwave a soup or ready-meal at lunch-time? If you don't feel full after eating one of these things, you can always supplement your lunch with fruit or a healthy snack.

Sometimes of course you might have a full cooked lunch. That's okay. On those days, why not eat a lighter evening meal than usual?

Dinner

In the previous chapter, I've already talked about a wide range of different foods, and how to choose lower calorie alternatives. You can use that information as a guide, when deciding what to eat for dinner.

The best dinners will be the ones that you prepare yourself using healthy low-calorie ingredients. When you start seriously thinking about what you eat, and what foods you buy, I expect you will discover (or rediscover) lots of tasty but healthy foods that would make a great dinner. In addition, if you ever get bored, you can keep your food interesting, but still low calorie, by experimenting with different sauces, spices, and condiments.

Finally, as I've said already, it is okay to have ready-meals and ready-prepared food once in a while, provided you choose the low calorie options. You really need to read those labels carefully!

Eating Out

Nearly all of us enjoying eating out from time-to-time, so I'm not going to suggest you abandon that – doing so would be too high in friction – and something you are unlikely to stick to. Instead, a better approach is to exercise care in your choice of restaurants, and in the dishes you choose when eating out.

1. Fast-food: If the food on the menu is all fried, as much as possible, I would suggest you simply avoid these restaurants completely – there's plenty of other restaurants you can go to. However, some fast-food chains have gradually improved, and offer some healthier options on their menus. Most of the large chains should also have a card or leaflet in their store which will tell you how many calories are in each of their dishes – study this information carefully. Generally speaking, I would suggest if you have a burger, having it without cheese, throwing away the bun (or half of it), avoiding French fries completely, and only drinking diet soda or water. Additionally, it is much better to eat grilled or oven-cooked chicken, rather

than fried chicken – and when you do eat chicken, be sure to cut off the skin. Also, you should be very careful of salads – the salad dressings, or pieces of fried chicken, etc., added to a salad, can add a huge number of calories!

2. Pizza: I don't suggest you eat pizza every day, but you can make it healthier than it otherwise would be, by having a thin-crust pizza (and especially avoiding stuffed crusts), asking for your pizza to be prepared without cheese, and instead adding flavour to your pizza by adding additional vegetable toppings.

3. Indian: When most people go to Indian restaurants, they eat lots of Indian breads, often prepared with ghee (Indian butter), fried foods such as samosas, pilau rice, and meat dishes too. This actually represents, in health terms, the worst of Indian cuisine (all the fried stuff and ghee), mixed with the worst Western influence (too much meat – many Indians in India either hardly eat meat or are complete vegetarians). However it's **easily** possible to have a very healthy Indian meal. First of all, cut out the fried stuff. Secondly, eat boiled/steamed rice instead of pilau rice or Indian bread (if you really must have bread, at least ask for it to be prepared without ghee). And thirdly, try eating less meat – if you look at the menu, or ask a waiter for advice, you should be able to find tons of very healthy vegetable dishes (just don't choose paneer, which is the Indian version of cheese).

4. Japanese: Japanese restaurants should be relatively easy to eat healthily at – there are lots of interesting dishes with soups, salads, grilled fish or meat, boiled rice, and of course sashimi (raw fish). Just avoid the fried stuff and the things coated in breadcrumbs ("panko").

5. Chinese: I've found a little harder to eat healthily at Chinese restaurants than at Japanese, but it is possible. Once again, the secret is to avoid the fried options (such as pancake rolls), choose boiled/steamed rice, and be sensible when selecting your main dish. Some Chinese restaurants also have an excellent selection of soups, which could be worth looking at.

6. Greek, Turkish, Persian, Lebanese, etc.: It's probably unfair of me to lump all these cuisines together, because they are different and distinct from each other, even though they share some similar dishes. That said, in most restaurants of this type, the "usual meal" is grilled meat accompanied by rice and/or unleavened bread. That's not so bad, provided you keep the portion size under control. Additionally, you don't have to go for the "usual meal" just because it is the obvious choice – have a proper look at the menu, and see if there are good lower-calorie options (for example grilled fish instead of red meat) available on the menu – you might also be pleasantly surprised at the vegetarian options that are available. Finally, my experience is that many Greek restaurants (including the ones in Cyprus) tend to serve some French fries with every meal – but

are more than happy to substitute a baked (jacket) potato if you ask them.

7. Other Cuisines: There numerous other types of restaurants and ethnic cuisines available, so I couldn't possibly try and discuss them all. You will have to use your good judgement and commonsense! As long as you are actually thinking about these issues when choosing your food, I'm sure you will get it right far more often than not.

Snacks

Lots of parents (and apparently some nutritionists) say that you shouldn't eat between meals. On the other hand, many nutritionists suggest that you should eat several small meals (basically snacks) per day, rather than just 2 or 3 large meals.

Frankly, as far as I am concerned, it doesn't matter who is right, because I personally find it impossible not to eat between meals. Keeping busy, and eating satisfying meals, does help me reduce the amount of snacking, but I know that I won't be able to eliminate the habit.

I've therefore come to conclusion that the best way to deal with snacking, is simply to keep some healthy and low-calorie snacks around (and conversely **not** to keep unhealthy high-calorie snacks around).

Here are some of the top items on my low-calorie snack-food list.

1. Fruit – Bananas, apples, oranges, and berries. You can also add other fruits as well to the list.

2. No-No Flat Breads – My calculation (using the hot 'n'spicy variety) tells me each individual cracker contains less than 30 calories. If you eat the spicy or herbed varieties, they are quite tasty (albeit a little dry) even on their own. Alternatively, you can use a low calorie topping such as ham, olive paste, or Gentlemen's Relish (a type of anchovy paste which you eat very sparingly). John West Dressed Crab or Lobster also makes a good topping – an entire 43g can, which is enough to cover quite a few crackers, is only about 61 calories (for crab), 45 calories (for lobster).

3. Matzo Crackers – Matzo crackers are also low calorie, and you can choose varieties with herb flavourings, and/or add your favourite low-calorie toppings. The ones that I eat, Rakusen's, are around 18 calories per cracker.

4. Rice Cakes – Again there are many different varieties to choose from. The cheapest ones from the local supermarket are 30 calories per large unsalted rice cake. I like to eat them with smoked salmon (which itself is only about 177 calories per 100g).

5. Cereal Bars – There are a huge range of different types of cereal bars on the market, and the amount of

calories per bar does vary widely, so you really need to read the labels carefully. Some bars can be less than 120 calories, whereas others are much more!

6. Cooked prawns (shrimp) or crayfish – A 125g packet of ready-to-eat prawns (shrimp) or crayfish is about 110 calories. I find it quite a satisfying snack. I often eat these accompanied with a small dollop of tomato ketchup or sweet chilli sauce, which does add a few extra calories, but makes the dish much tastier.

7. Pickled Mussels or Cockles – Pickled mussels or cockles in vinegar are also quite low calorie, and a fairly satisfying snack. The jar of cockles that I am looking at right now weighs 200g including the vinegar, and has a drained weight of 90g. The calories are expressed per 100g of drained weight, so it took a bit of figuring out: I make it 105 calories that I would actually consume if I drained the jar and then ate all the cockles.

8. Pickled Mushrooms: I discovered these by chance in the Polish section of a local supermarket (this kind of discovery is exactly why it's a good idea to go down every aisle in the supermarket when shopping), and they make an excellent snack. The variety that I buy comes in 300g jars and contains two suggested servings – half a jar is 65 calories, and a whole jar (which is quite a lot mushrooms) is just 130 calories!

9. Corn on the cob – around 100 calories for a medium corn cob. Do **not** add butter – each tablespoon of

butter adds another 100 calories! Instead, I suggest you learn to love your corn plain (fresh corn really is quite tasty), but if you really must add something try lemon juice (only 4 calories per tablespoon) and/or a little chilli powder.

10. A couple of cooked beetroots from a vacuum pack – around 50 calories.

11. Mange Tout – Wash, throw it in a bowl when still damp, and microwave. An entire 180g packet (which is rather a lot to eat in one sitting) is less than 70 calories.

Of course, the above are just suggestions to get you started – once you start really looking around when shopping, I'm sure you will be able to find many more low calorie snack options that you will enjoy eating.

Other Tips

Here are some other weight loss tips that I've picked up along the way. I can't guarantee that they all work – all I can say is that I have personally tried them all!

1. High Intensity Interval Training (HIIT)

The idea here is that supposedly doing short bursts of intense exercise, separated by less-intensive recovery periods, is supposedly a better at producing results than exercising at a steady rate. There's a Wikipedia page about this at http://en.wikipedia.org/wiki/High-intensity_interval_training.

If you want to try this, you want to be sure you don't push yourself too hard (talk to your doctor first!), especially if you've got an existing medical condition, or if you're extremely unfit, or if you are just getting on in years. The last thing you want to do is to cause a heart-attack or do yourself an injury.

Anyway, I have experimented with an amateur "homemade" version of HIIT:

(i) When running, I usually do laps round a small local recreation ground. It's probably 200m per side, so an entire lap is about 800m. My "homemade" version of HIIT is to sprint one of the sides as fast as I can.

(ii) When swimming, I normally swim a steady front-crawl. However, my "homemade" version of HIIT is to swim every fourth lap as fast as I possibly can.

(iii) When riding the static exercise bike, I try and speed up during the adverts, or at least 1 or 2 minutes in each 10.

To be honest, I haven't been as diligent as I should have been in maintaining these habits on a consistent basis, so I haven't benefited nearly as much as I should. Nevertheless, when I have done these things, I have felt the difference after just a few days – sprinting 200 metres in the middle of a long run quickly goes from being absolutely exhausting to being relatively easy.

2. Swimming in the Sea

The first time I was set to do the Bournemouth to Boscombe swim, I was quite worried. I had spent a lot of time swimming in the pool, but swimming in the sea is very different.

My home in England is nowhere near the sea (I actually live just about the furthest point from the sea possible on this island), but I was able to get lots of practice in by swimming in the sea, every single day, when on vacation in Cyprus.

After the vacation, I returned to England, and weighed myself for the first time in two weeks. I was actually dreading the result – I had probably eaten more than I should, and hadn't really taken any exercise other than swimming for about 1 hour per day. I was however surprised to learn I had actually lost 7 pounds!

Your experience may vary, but on thinking about it, I have to say there is a lot to be said for regular sea swimming. Quite apart from the exercise you get from the swimming, even a warm sea is usually colder than the swimming pool, and you will burn quite a few calories just maintaining your body temperature. When I was swimming in Cyprus, the sea temperature was around 24 degrees Celsius at the time, whereas the swimming pool at my local sports centre is maintained at approximately 29 degrees Celsius.

I am **not** of course suggesting that your swim beyond your abilities, take silly risks, or give yourself hypothermia by staying too long in cold water. Obviously you have to be sensible about these things. What I can say is that I **never** swam beyond my comfort zone, and **never** felt cold swimming in Cyprus.

3. Cold Showers

Cold showers supposedly increase your metabolic rate. I don't know if it's true or not, but I have tried it – it's certainly invigorating, and not at all unpleasant.

However, I find it virtually impossible to step under a

freezing cold shower, and I expect you might too. There's a trick however that you can use to easily get a cold shower:

(i) At the end of your normal shower, while standing under the main stream of water, turn the tap halfway towards cold. It will be quite a shock for a moment, but after a few seconds, you should get used to it.

(ii) Still standing up the main stream of water, now turn the tap all the way towards cold. Again, you will feel a shock, but again it will seem quite normal after a few seconds.

Using this technique, it really isn't difficult to have a 30 second or 1 minute cold shower.

4. Keep Reading, Learning & Listening

During my weight loss journey, I read a lot, especially online, about health, fitness, and weight loss.. Of course, I always remained cautious when reading about weight loss claims, especially from people hawking products or services, but even so, I can certainly say that I learned quite a few things

Some of the information helped me directly. Other information helped me to maintain my motivation, or provided me with greater insight. So, I can definitely say it was a worthwhile activity.

I couldn't possibly remember every website that I visited, but the most memorable one was a course that I bought called "The Truth About Six Pack Abs" (you will find a link to it on my website at http://www.suniltanna.com/weightloss). No, I haven't got six packs abs, as much as I might wish for them, but I have picked up lots of interesting ideas from the product itself, and from the author's email newsletter.

More generally speaking, I'm always on the look-out for new ideas to improve my diet, get more exercise, and increase my metabolism (so my body burns more calories), and you should be too.

Epilogue

It took me more than 2 years to do it, but I got rid of the flab, and radically improved my fitness.

I feel much better. I enjoy regular sport, and have participated in exciting challenges such as cross-country running races, the Bournemouth to Boscombe sea swim, and the Nuts Challenge (a cross-country assault course), however none of these are the most important or exciting thing about my life.

The biggest and most exciting news is the arrival of my son Byron, who was born in December 2011, but that's another story...

Here's a picture of my family at the Bournemouth-Boscombe swim in 2012.

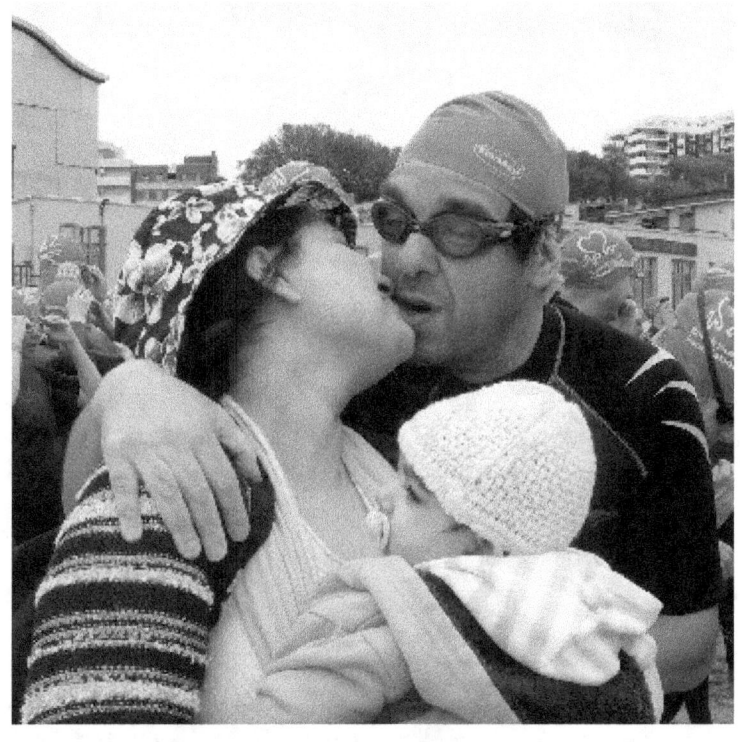

You can keep up with my latest news at
http://www.suniltanna.com/weightloss

www.ingramcontent.com/pod-product-compliance
Lightning Source LLC
Chambersburg PA
CBHW070611290526
45790CB00002B/878